Engraved

By Alma Bemis

*(Hebrews 10:16 NIV) "This is the covenant I will make with them after that time, says the Lord. I will put my laws in their **hearts**, and I will write them on their **minds.**"*
(Jeremiah 31:33b NIV) also adds: "I will be their God, and they will be my people

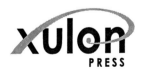

Copyright © 2009 by Alma Bemis

Engraved
by Alma Bemis

Printed in the United States of America

ISBN 978-1-60791-106-7

All rights reserved solely by the author. The author guarantees all contents are original and do not infringe upon the legal rights of any other person or work. No part of this book may be reproduced in any form without the permission of the author. The views expressed in this book are not necessarily those of the publisher.

Unless otherwise indicated, Bible quotations are taken from The King James Version, and The New International Version, Copyright © 1973, 1978, 1984 by International Bible Society/The Zondervan Bible Publishers, and The New Revised Standard Version, Copyright © 1989 by Division of Christian Education of the National Counsel of the Churches of Christ.

www.xulonpress.com

Forward

ENGRAVED IS THE STORY OF A VERY EXCITING AND CHALLENGING SPIRITUAL JOURNEY. It is always exciting to take a journey. The problem with a spiritual journey is that they have high mountains, and sometimes very deep valleys That is exactly what I experienced and you will experience in reading the story of Alma Bemis' spiritual journey in her new manuscript, Engraved. What I did not expect is that I, too, would experience the high and low emotions as I read the book. Alma, in her delightful way with words, takes us with her into the highs and lows of her personal spiritual journey.

I have always known Alma Bemis as a woman of faith, even when she was a child. However, I never really knew the depth of her faith until I read her book. The devastating news of inoperable cancer that she received must have come to her as something that she could not believe. Yet it was true, Alma had cancer, and if there was not a miracle, it could be the end of a very productive and anointed life. But, Alma decided to believe.

I knew this great woman of faith well enough to know that she would respond in faith, but I was not prepared for the depth of faith that she would demonstrate even when most people would have chosen to give up. I remember going to her home and seeing the walls, the refrigerator, even the windows with scriptures declaring who she was in God. Everywhere you looked you saw faith. And that is the way it is with the book, no matter how bad the news, no matter how impossible the circumstance, or how high the mountain, Alma chose to respond to the impossible with a faith that could not be destroyed.

And that is the very reason this book is a journey. It is the story of a woman, who stands head and shoulders above almost every other believer that never sees the impossibility of the valley, but rather the wonder of the mountain. It is the journey of a woman who was physically in a deep, impossible valley, but spiritually she leads us from the mountaintop of faith.

If you are living in an impossible circumstance, if you have ever lived through an impossible circumstance, or if you have lived in a faith that has never been challenged, you need to read "ENGRAVED". Yes, it will inspire you, but most of all it will challenge you. For everyone, you need this book. In fact, never have I ever seen faith so radically and magnificently described as I hear it in this manuscript.

So, I invite you to take this journey with me. If you do, I know you will want to pass it on to someone who is facing a severe spiritual crisis. Come; take a journey with me into the wonder of a world where nothing is impossible.

Rev. Thomas F. Reid / Senior Pastor/The Tabernacle/ Orchard Park, NY 14127

Introduction

Here it is almost 4:30 am, and I am so full I had to get up and start this book.

Months ago Shawn, one of the Elders of Family Worship Center, asked me a question; "What is the title to your book?" I sort of chuckled because I had just shared with the Elders and their spouses, another aspect of my testimony, and that was his response. At that moment I said, probably, "The Lord is My Shepherd". Tonight, I realized that God has given me five chapter titles that are engraved in my heart and mind forever. As you continue to read, my prayer is that the Holy Spirit will take what has been engraved in my heart, and make it so real to you, that you will have a fresh revelation of the love God has for your life, no matter what valley you are walking through. My present valley just happens to be cancer. I know that it affects every fiber of your being. It must be dealt with body, soul and spirit. Many people give cancer a capital C, but in reality it is lower case. I KNOW Christ is the one whose name is above all names, including cancer.

Dedication

I first want to dedicate this book to
God the Father who has loved me with
Immeasurable-Unconditional Love.
Jesus Christ, my Great High Priest, who
not only prays for me, but actually bore my
iniquities and disease in His own body, that I
can receive His promise:
"By His stripes I am healed."
And The Holy Spirit, whose guidance and
power continues to lead me safely through
this incredible journey called life.

Second, I can't say enough about my
husband David
who has stood with me through the fire.
He was there for every test, surgery, chemo,
or radiation treatment.
His standing in faith means the world to me.

Thirdly, even though there have been many doctors and medical people involved in this process...three of them have walked with me in this journey with such compassion and professionalism I can't help but say thank you to them and all their colleagues connected with McGee's.Women's Hospital of Pittsburgh,PA and
The Regional Cancer Center of Erie, PA.
Dr. Krivak, my Oncologist
Dr. Barriwall, my Radiologist
Dr. Sagan, my Urologist

Fourth, to Mike and Debbie Griesbaum, who went the second mile with me, in the middle of their walk of faith. Mike just had a heart transplant after 5 years of living with only one artery working.
I proudly call them, "My Partners in Faith."

Fifth, to Darlene, Radhica, and Mary Jo who made my day to day walk so much easier; just through their countless deeds of love.

Sixth, to David, Heather, Todd, Maria, Jacob and Hannah my precious gifts from God who have stood by their Mom and Grandma during our journey of faith.
I love you, and pray that God will multiply faith to each of you.

Seventh to Julie Alvarez for dedicating her talents to this book.

Eight, to Pastor Reid and Wanda, my spiritual parents, and all my family and friends who have been standing in faith with me throughout the world. Your letters, prayers, and even gifts of love have encouraged me to go forward with expectation.

Thank you.

Chapter 1.	Perfect Peace	17
Chapter 2.	Grace in Tribulation	31
Chapter 3.	The Lord is My Shepherd	47
Chapter 4.	The Banqueting Table	61
Chapter 5.	Today	69

Perfect Peace

—⋘—

Every year I ask God to give me a Word to meditate on throughout the year. In 2006, the Word was "Perfect Peace."

In May of that year, I called my family doctor's office and asked for a referral to a bladder specialist, because I felt like my insides were falling out. The specialist scheduled a test for June 19th, to determine my bladder's capacity to function properly. He told me that my bladder was fine, that I needed to lose weight; exercise to strengthen that part of my body, and that probably some of the pain which I was feeling was my sciatic nerve. He also told me that he could probably help me. I figured that if what he said was true, I would go to my chiropractor for decompression therapy, and start on a diet to lose weight.

My chiropractor is a wonderful man and started decompression therapy, but recommended that I get an MRI. He could not order it, because my insurance did not recognize him. I began to feel much better, so I did not request the MRI from my family doctor. (My mistake was I should have gone to my family doctor in the first place. He would have ordered the necessary test before he sent me to the bladder specialist.)

I went for therapy from June until October, and was feeling much better. The chiropractor reduced my schedule for treatments from three days a week to one day a week. During the last three weeks of treatments, I began to feel worse. I told him, and he told me that he could no longer treat me without an MRI. He also told me to give my back a rest.

I went to my family doctor, on 11/21, he ordered test, and referred me back to the urologist. The test showed that there was a problem with my urethra between by kidney and bladder. I went to the urologist on December 18th, and he scheduled further testing for the middle of January.

For some strange reason, I did not feel content with waiting for that test. Then I began to bleed, and felt that I needed to contact a gynecologist. I was told that they were not accepting new patients before the beginning of the year. I had a total hysterectomy in 1994, and never sought out a gynecologist after I moved to Erie in 1999. I thought I would be fine with just a family doctor. I figured, what's two more weeks, I'll call back in January. When I did, even though I told them again about the hysterectomy and bleeding, I was now told that I could not get an appointment before March or April. I received the same response from calling several offices.

Enough is enough with no real answers! I decided that I could no longer wait, so I called my family doctor's office and requested that he do an internal. He did, and when he did, he said, "Oh my word, you have a mass!" When he spoke that out to me, peace came over me. I knew I was in God's hands and now I could go forward and deal with the real problem. He immediately sent me up for pre-op test, so I would be prepared for surgery. He also connected me with a local gynecologist.

PEACE!!!

How in the world could I have peace, when I was just told that I have a mass? Well, I had been meditating all year on the Word, "Perfect Peace" When peace hit me; I knew I was in the palm of God's hand. The peace that came is described in the Bible.

(Phillippians 4:6 – 7 NIV) Do not be anxious about anything, but in everything, by prayer and petition, with thanksgiving, present your requests to God. And the peace of God, which transcends all understanding, will guard your hearts and your minds in Christ Jesus.

Trust me when I say, I had already been in prayer...but years of God's faithfulness had produced in me a heart of trust in Him.

Let me give you a few examples:

I was the second youngest of 15 children. My younger twin brother died several weeks after our birth. Often growing up, I would wonder, why did he die, and not me? But then I accepted Jesus Christ as my personal Savior, at seven years of age, while attending Bible School, at Hillview Baptist Church. To be honest with you, I don't remember if I was attending Vacation Bible School or a Bible Club. I don't even remember how I got there. Most of my family, in general, was not even attending church. I just know where I was when Christ came into my heart. From that moment on, a new journey developed. It was a journey of discovering God's love and purpose for my life.

It was shortly after that, a gentleman by the name of Mr. Hopkins came to our home and offered to drive those of us that wanted to go to Sunday school, to a local Assembly of God church. Several of us started to attend, and I fell in love with learning the truth in the Bible. There was something wonderful about Father God who loved me so much that He sent His Son to die for my sins, so I could be one of His children. It was a child-like faith that just accepted that incredible love. I will always be grateful for that faith, because the years ahead could have embittered me to any relationship to a father.

My father was an alcoholic, and as I grew, I watched what alcohol could do to destroy a family. I won't get into the destruction part in this book, but I will tell you this much, I serve an awesome God that not only loved me, but He also loved my entire family, including my dad.

When I was a teenager, attending South Buffalo Tabernacle, I remember praying at the altar. I don't know what kind of prayer you would call it, but I was desperately crying out to God to save my dad. I knew his salvation would affect my family's future. Rev. Albert Reid didn't know what I was praying about, but he encouraged me to not beg God, but to trust Him. At that moment a seed of faith was planted in my heart. I went through times of tears as a teenager, over the affects of alcohol, but something inside of me knew my dad would not die before finding Christ as his Savior.

I remember one night, alone in my bedroom, reading:

(Psalms 56:8 NRSV) You have kept count of my tossings; put my tears in your bottle. Are they not in your record?

I realized how important my tears where to God. He knew what I was going through. He saw the sleepless nights. He heard the screaming. He saw me tossing and turning in my bed. He didn't take me out of my circumstances...but He did help me to grow in the midst of them.

Two great aspects of that growth came when I was twelve years old. One was the Baptism in the Holy Spirit, and the other was a dream to become a Pastor's wife. That dream, and the power of The Holy Spirit kept me focused on my future, not the present circumstances.

I was around 20 years of age when my faith for my dad's salvation was challenged. The doctors told us that my father was dying. They said that if he did live, he would end up in a vegetated state at a nursing home. He would never return home! I remember standing against the wall in the hospital room, staring at him. What a wasted life! Fifteen beautiful children that he could of enjoyed, but because he could not forgive people in his past, he lived a life most of us would have regretted.

There he lay barely able to communicate. Food was caught in his mouth, and his eyes would hardly open. He could not even stand on his feet. My husband stood at his side talking to Him, and I silently stood against the wall talking to God. "Father, I believed you all these years, now I need the evidence!" As soon as I prayed that prayer, I heard my husband say, "Dad, where's Jesus?" As clear as clear can be, he said, "He's in my heart." Within the week, my dad was totally healed, and completely set free from alcohol. The next time I saw my dad, he was at home, dressing and feeding himself. He entered his own new journey that lasted another seven years on this earth, but is lasting for eternity in the presence of God.

When my daughter Heather was in the eight grade; she came home from school and told me that her gums hurt. She always had perfect teeth, but I immediately scheduled her to see our dentist. He put her on an antibiotic and rescheduled her to come back. When we went back, he looked at me and told me to get my daughter to my family doctor immediately. There is something seriously wrong with her that has nothing to do with her teeth. She had been complaining that other parts of her body were beginning to hurt.

When I took her to our family doctor, he immediately put her in the hospital, and began a series of test. All the tests were coming back negative, except the pain was getting worse and worse. Heather was diagnosed with childhood rheumatoid arthritis. The pain was so severe in all of her joints; we had to wrap them in ice. The doctors told me that she would be on heavy medication the rest of her life, that could cause serious problems to her stomach, and she probably would end up in a wheel chair. Not only was she in pain, but because of the attack on the joints, she became severely anemic.

But God!

We prayed, we believed, and she grabbed hold of faith. There would be times she would lay in her bed, and instead of screaming out with pain, she would begin to sing. I was amazed at some of the hymns she had memorized. I won't get into all the diagnosis, or possible causes, but I will shout the song of victory! In less than a year she was totally off all medication, and free from arthritis, plus now able to play soccer.

In these few paragraphs, I have shared that God is a God of love, salvation, empowerment, dreams, deliverance and healing. By the way, my husband is a Pastor; so you can see God's call to a twelve year old was right on.

Peace isn't something that just happens. Peace develops out of relationship to a loving God.

(Isaiah 26:3 NIV) You will keep in perfect peace him whose mind is steadfast, because he trusts in you.

Jesus told us that He gives us peace.

(John 14:27 NIV) Peace I leave with you; my peace I give you. I do not give to you as the world gives. Do not let your hearts be troubled and do not be afraid.

The only way you can know real peace in the midst of your storms is to become a part of His kingdom.

(Romans 14:17 NIV) For the kingdom of God is not a matter of eating and drinking, but of righteousness, peace and joy in the Holy Spirit,

However, you can't even come into His kingdom without accepting the Prince of Peace.

(Isaiah 9:6 NIV) For to us a child is born, to us a son is given, and the government will be on his shoulders. And he will be called Wonderful Counselor, Mighty God, Everlasting Father, Prince of Peace.

(John 14:6 NIV) Jesus answered, "I am the way and the truth and the life. No one comes to the Father except through me.

Nicodemus was a Jewish Rabbi who was asking Jesus questions about God. This is Jesus' answer;

(John 3:3 NIV) In reply Jesus declared, "I tell you the truth, no one can see the kingdom of God unless he is <u>born again</u>."

What does it mean to be born again? You must first recognize that you are a sinner, and that you have need of a Savior.

(Romans 3:23 NIV) for all have sinned and fall short of the glory of God,

You must believe that Jesus paid the penalty for your sin.

(Isaiah 53:5 -6 NIV) But he was pierced for our transgressions, he was crushed for our iniquities; the punishment that brought us peace was upon him, and by his wounds we are healed. We all, like sheep, have gone astray, each of us has turned to his own way; and the LORD has laid on him the iniquity of us all.

Now you must speak it with your mouth, and believe it with your heart.

(Romans 10:9 NIV) That if you confess with your mouth, "Jesus is Lord," and believe in your heart that God raised him from the dead, you will be saved.

If you haven't done it yet...do it now! There is nothing else in this world that can give you God's wonderful peace.

Here's a simple prayer to help.

Father:

You know everything about my life; the good and the bad. Yet you said that you loved me and gave your Son Jesus to die on the cross for my sins. I accept His sacrifice for my sins as an act of your love. Forgive me of my sins, and from this moment on, created in me a clean heart and a right spirit that hungers to know you more. Lead my steps to a place where I can grow in your love. Thank You.

Father:

I want to thank you that I discovered the Prince of Peace at the age of seven, and He has never left me or forsaken me. I want to thank you that when I was told that I had a mass, you covered me in peace. You reminded me that I was in the palm of your hand. You reminded me that you healed my father and my daughter. Through many years I have seen your faithfulness, watched you order my steps, and calm my heart. I want to thank you that I can trust you, because through multiple storms of life…You have been there, holding, teaching, guiding, and strengthening me day by day.

Grace in Tribulation

—m—

On Wednesday, January 17, 2007, my husband and I left home to visit the gynecologist. I first was scheduled for a sonogram, and then went in to see the doctor. As soon as he examined me, he told me he had bad news. I told him I wanted to get my husband. When he came in to see us his words were that I had an inoperable-cancerous tumor. He also told me that I would have to go to a gynecological oncologist and that there were none in Erie. He set up an appointment for me to go to McGee Women's Hospital in Pittsburgh, PA, for the 22nd. The hospital is about two hours from our home.

We both were sort of quiet on the way home. I realized that I could not just have surgery to remove this tumor. I felt a tear fall down my face, and I just asked God, "How do I tell people?" His immediate answer to me was incredible. He told me to "Tell people to tell you five things you are in Me."

I walked in our home and saw my son, Todd. At the time I was watching my grandson, Jacob while Maria and Todd worked. Todd stayed home with

Jacob until I returned home. I walked in the house, saw him, and asked him to tell me five things I was in Christ. He started: (I added the Scripture references for your benefit.)

> **You are the apple of His Eye.** (Psalms 17:8 NIV) *Keep me as the apple of your eye; hide me in the shadow of your wings*
> **You are more than a conqueror.** *(Rom 8:37 NIV) No, in all these things we are more than conquerors through him who loved us.*
> **You are the righteousness of God.** *(2 Cor 5:21 NIV) God made him who had no sin to be sin for us, so that in him we might become the righteousness of God.*
> **You are healed by His stripes.** *(Isaiah 53:5 KJV) But he was wounded for our transgressions, he was bruised for our iniquities: the chastisement of our peace was upon him; and with his stripes we are healed.*
> **You're an over comer** *(Rev 12:11 NIV) They overcame him by the blood of the Lamb and by the word of their testimony; they did not love their lives so much as to shrink from death.*

I looked Todd straight in the eyes and told him to remember that what he had just spoken was God's view. Now I'm going to tell you the bird's eye view, and the bird happens to be a vulture. But, I want you to remember God's view whenever you are thinking about me. An incredible thing happened in those moments of sharing with people throughout the day. As the Word was spoken, not only was I strengthened, but so were the people telling me who I was in Christ. Their focus became God's ability to heal me, rather than the enemy's ability to destroy me.

(John 10:10 KJV) The thief cometh not, but for to steal, and to kill, and to destroy: I am come that they might have life, and that they might have it more abundantly.

I want to share a little funny story with you. We had lived in our present home for over seven years, and until now, I never had wild turkeys in my yard. Now I was having about 23 of them on a regular basis. They aren't the prettiest bird in the world. Sometimes I thought they looked a little like vultures. Going through my present circumstances, I almost felt like the enemy was sending the birds in my yard to mock me.

One day, as I was looking at them, I decided to think of turkeys in connection to Thanksgiving. When I did, I realized that every time I saw them, I was going to think of things I was thankful for. What a difference it made. When they came, I gave thanks, and began to laugh. Shortly after my breakthrough they stopped coming regularly. They still come occasionally, but now I look forward to a time of thanksgiving and laughter.

The next day, we received word that a member of our congregation's sister was in the hospital dying. As we went to the hospital two of the women in

Engraved

leadership were already with the family. They came and sat by me. As we shared, I thought about how I would tell the rest of my women. I knew I had scheduled a Women's Night Out on Friday evening, so I asked them to please prepare a banqueting table on the platform for Friday night. Make it as beautiful as you can. Then I asked Karen if she would make little place setting cards that declared things that we have access to at the banqueting table. The girls readily agreed to do the assignment. This was going to be my way of telling the women about the cancer. I had a special speaker coming, but I did not share with her what was going on ahead of time.

Lenny, one of our Elders, called on Thursday and told us that the Elders were coming to his house for prayer. I want all of you to know that about a year earlier, Lenny's wife went home to be with the Lord, after her battle with cancer. Before Debbie died, our Women's ministry made no-sew blankets for women in the church that were going through battles. I asked the women to wrap them around the women and tell them that every time they put the blanket on themselves to remember that the Holy Spirit was covering them, and people were praying for them. Lenny took Debbie's blanket and wrapped it around me that night. Then he handed me a Scripture verse:

(Psalms 117:1-2 KJV) O Praise the LORD, all ye nations: praise him, all ye people. For his merciful kindness is great toward us: and the truth of the LORD endureth for ever. Praise ye the LORD.

All our Elders where there to encourage us and do battle through prayer. It was a powerful night.

Our son, Todd saw a vision, and began to share it with us. He said he saw Jesus walking around me, with His eyes continuously fixed on the tumor. I immediately remembered the Scripture in Revelation:

(Rev 2:18 NIV) "To the angel of the church in Thyatira write: These are the words of the Son of God, whose eyes are like blazing fire and whose feet are like burnished bronze.

When I was teaching the Book of Revelation to our women, I would tell them that Jesus was presenting Himself as the answer to the problems He was seeing in churches, before He presented the problems. In this church there was a Jezebel spirit that brought deception into the church. I explained to them, that if we allow Him to look with His flaming eyes into our hearts on a regular basis, he would deal with our offenses, so Jezebel would not have a hold on us. Now those same eyes were looking at my tumor, and I knew, that if I continued to trust Him, those same eyes that could cleanse my heart of all impurities, could certainly deal with this cancer.

The brass feet reminded me of when they used brass in the Old Testament to make the laver for the Tabernacle. The brass shone like a mirror, and showed the need for cleansing through the washing of the Word.

(Eph 5:25- 26 KJV) Husbands, love your wives, even as Christ also loved the church, and gave himself for it; that he might sanctify and cleanse it with the washing of water by the word,

I believe that as we allow Him to cleanse our hearts through the washing of the Word, we will have feet that will take His peace with us wherever we go.

Friday night came and I asked the Women's leadership to get there early for prayer. I also asked them to set up a gossip table by the altar. I wanted three of the women to sit there and just gossip about someone who had just received a negative report. We had prayer, and the building started to fill up with women from all over. There were probably over 70 women. I couldn't wait to start. The table was beautiful, my gossipers were ready, and I was full of the Word. About two minutes before 7 PM, I got up and found myself saying. "In His presence there is fullness of joy." I did not know that the Lord changed the speaker's message, and told her to speak on

(Psalms 16:11 KJV) Thou wilt show me the path of life: in thy presence is fullness of joy; at thy right hand there are pleasures for evermore.

There were people from Anita McCoy's church, including her Pastor's wife, Lady Jones. There were also leaders from Women Aglow. I was thrilled, but I knew only God could turn our sorrow to dancing that night. I asked my gossipers to do their unprompted skit. I didn't know quite what to expect. Theresa started with, "Did you hear that Mary Smith had a heart attack, and the doctors told her she most likely will not survive." "I agree! " Darlene, stood up, and began to speak. "Don't you know that the power of life and death is in your tongue?" She just went to town. She told me later, she didn't even see Theresa, but she felt to do battle against the words that were spoken. It was perfect!

I got up and told the crowd the report that I had received three days earlier. Then I saw Judy in the back of the church. Judy had been going through chemo this last year to deal with severe hepatitis of the liver. I went back, grabbed her hand, and said, "Come on Sweetie, you and I are going to the banqueting table." Then I had the girls come up and pick out a place card that showed them something that was available for them at the table. They began to speak them out...laughter, healing, peace, joy, boldness, etc. There were over seventy things available. They got it!

The wonderful thing is that several months later, Judy came back with a report from her doctor. He had asked her what she was doing different. She told him the only thing was prayer. He told her to keep it up because her liver was healing itself.

I recently read an anonymous saying:

"Peace is not the absence of trouble.
Peace is the presence of God."

Engraved

It was a humbling night as Anita and Lady Jones began to minister to me. They began to pray that I would be able to walk through this valley to victory. After the service was over, and my husband returned, several of them asked if they could pray for the both of us. They just began to prophesy over us. They said that we would be one flesh. They said that we would share the pulpit. There was so much, I can't even remember it all, but those two things stood out to me.

Again, Sunday, the people had a time of prayer over me.

When I woke up for prayer on Monday morning, the Lord spoke to me. He did not want me doing battle; He just wanted me to rest in Him. Earlier in the week He told me that I would have times that I would be building myself up in the Lord, times I would be wondering if He had deserted me, and times that I would KNOW who I AM in Him. In all of those times, He would still love me. He doesn't just love me when I've got it all together, He loves me when I am weak, and when I am strong.

I would awake with songs in my heart like…"It is Finished", "Jesus, Jesus, Lord to Me", and many others. What a way to wake up.

I arrived in Pittsburgh that day, and met Dr. Krivak for the very first time. Because the Hospital is a teaching facility, there were others with him. He took one look at the tumor and said something like "Oh my…this is bigger than me; I need to call others in."

The next thing I knew was that there were about six doctors in the room. They were very international, and I told them so. Yet in the back of my mind I remembered the Scripture that Lenny had given me Thursday night.

(Psalms 117:1 -2 NIV) Praise the LORD, all you nations; extol him, all you peoples. For great is his love toward us, and the faithfulness of the LORD endures forever. Praise the LORD.

I looked at them, thinking they would be part of the nations praising Him.

Mike and Debbie Griesbaum had driven down with us that day. Mike was waiting for a heart transplant, and both Mike and Debbie were able to speak to us in ways no one else could. They had been walking through their battle for five years. Another couple was going to go with us, but I know God designed that day for us to be with Mike and Debbie.

I was immediately admitted, and the test began shortly after. Let me say the next few days were full of tests and questions. I had biopsies, catheters, blood test, EKG, sonograms, cat scans, pet/cat scan combination, bladder and kidney test, IV's, anesthesia twice in one day. I even went home at the end of the week radio-active for 48 hours. They determined that I had a vaginal tumor that was glandular. That was strange in of itself, because the vaginal area is not a gland. They began to share with me the treatments that I would have to go through up at the Regional Cancer

Engraved

Center in Erie. It was a combination of both radiation and chemo therapy.

Before I went to McGee, I prayed about going to another facility that treated you body, soul, and spirit. The Lord told me no. I want you at McGee. Let me tell you I was surrounded by people of faith, and three incredible doctors. Trust me; none of the staff at the hospital abused their rights to speak about God to me. I was the one who always brought the subject up. It opened the door for them to speak. It was incredible, because I spoke to technicians, people in recovery, people transporting me, and the nurses. When they would ask me how I was doing, I would say, "I'm in the palm of God's hand." Boy did that open the door to testimonies, and conversations.

The very first nurse assigned to me, responded by telling me her story. She had tumors on her ovaries, and went in for surgery to have the ovaries removed. When she woke up, she had no pain, and inquired of the doctor. He told her the tumors were gone, and they did not have to do surgery. She was excited and very pregnant as she shared the good report with me.

Another nurse in the recovery area began to share with me her faith in God as she was battling with cancer. She sought me out later and gave me Dodie Osteen's book…"Healed of Cancer".

One nurse seeing me going into surgery for biopsies gave me a kiss and told me she was praying for me.

Norman, a young man who would often transported me for test; began to tell me more things I was in Christ, after I told him I was in the palm of God's hand, and the apple of His eye. It was wonderful having him transport me, watching his friendliness to staff and others throughout the hospital. I will never forget his name, because my twin brother had the same name. He told me that they knew I was going through a tough time, but I was always encouraging them.

One of the nurses asked if I minded if Sister Nora who was a catholic nun and the chaplain at the hospital, visit me. I told her I would be glad to have her come. We had a wonderful time together sharing about the Lord. She prayed a prayer over me that included rooting out every cancer cell in my body.

Another nurse who had to explain a particular procedure to me asked if she could pray for both, my husband and I. Then she shared she would have her church pray for us, with our permission.

A young man, who was helping transport me to my car, handed me a poem, in the elevator, that he had just written. That poem was about drawing close to God. I thanked him, and encouraged him to continue to write. What a way to leave a hospital!

It was amazing to me, out of all the workers in the hospital, how God surrounded me with people of faith. Not all were, but enough to make a difference in my valley.

A few years ago, I was on my way to Buffalo, to go with my daughter Heather for some test. On my way up, I began to sing. This was my new song.

**Even though it feels like defeat Lord
Your resurrection power is near.
Even though it feels like death itself
Your message is very clear.
Your power is greater than sin Lord.
Your power is greater than disease.
Your power is greater than death itself,
And Your power is living in me.
Your power brings victory.**

Heather's test results were fine. Let me tell you, the reality of that song rang in my ears during my current battle. His power brings victory. When a nurse came into my room she told me that the doctors were in consultation with each other about me. I was reminded of the power that brings victory, and I began to pray in the Spirit for those doctors. I know the one doctor was frustrated because he was going to have to send me home with out the entire test being completed. The frustration is now having to deal with doctors who are not a part of the team, and scheduling appointments. Before the day was over one test was completed, and the others were being scheduled for the beginning of next week.

As I returned the following Monday, I continued to feed myself the Word which told me who I was in Christ. I would listen to and sing songs that just would well up in my soul. God spoke to my heart and told me on Tuesday "You are going to hear more than what you want to hear, but trust me." Later in that day, two of the doctors came into my room to tell me that they may have to change the treatment plan because I may have fourth-stage cancer. I asked them what that meant. They told me that it looked like the cancer had spread to other parts of my body, including my lungs. They were now going to have to do a needle biopsy of the lungs to determine what they were seeing.

I looked at the doctor and asked him, how long he thought I had to live. He told me that he couldn't tell me that. 'First of all you are young and healthy, and second of all you have faith.'

I asked him to tell me what the average was; because I didn't want to lie around in a hospital if I was going to die...I wanted to live everyday that I had left. He told me 4 to 6 months, but then told me that they are not sure there was cancer in my lungs, and they were going to do everything they could to extend my life and bring a cure. I asked him if I could pray for him. I took his hand and began to pray for wisdom. The other doctor, asked me to pray for direction.

When I was getting my sonogram, I told the technician that God has given me peace, and I was going to stay in the palm of His hand. She told me that it was great, because so many people try to stay in control of their own situations, when they have no control. That's it, isn't it...God is in control. He knows the plans He has for me. He holds up a standard against the enemy. He gives me peace in the midst of the storm. He walks me through the valley of the shadow of death. He is my strength and song. He is my deliverer. I can't control the days ahead, but I certainly know who does.

Engraved

One day I asked my husband what the number five meant. He told me GRACE. Later when I was sharing with Tyanne Jurka, missionary to Honduras, she said yes but its Grace in Tribulation. I laugh because God could have given me any number…but instead He chose five things you are in Christ. Why? Because He knew if I could get it in my spirit, I would have the grace that I needed to get through the months ahead.

Engraved

Father:

You are so awesome. You knew what I needed before I even came to you. Not only did you want to build up my spirit, but you used;

> Your Written Word,
> Your Spoken Word,
> Words of Songs,
> and
> Words of Testimonies.
> Thank You
> for
> Words of life.

The Lord is My Shepherd

In 2006, Rev. Gary Kellner spoke at our church. He was presently reaching out to the nation of Ukraine. As he shared about the plight of many of the women, my heart began to think of Pastor Gwen Mouliet of Pamona, NJ. I knew in my spirit that she would be the perfect person to speak into the lives of these Ukrainian women. Darlene, one of the women from our church, having a Russian heritage, had asked if she could join us for lunch. She could not get these women off her heart. I told Gary about Pastor Gwen, and asked if he would be interested in her speaking at the Women's Conferences they were setting up throughout Ukraine. He said he would be delighted to have her be part of the team going over.

I called Gwen, and she was in one of the Virginia's ministering at a Woman's Conference. She didn't have time to talk. I said, I just wanted to ask her one question, and she could get back to me. I proceeded to ask her if she was willing to go to Ukraine. She asked me if that was Russia. I said it use to be a part

Engraved

of it. She began to tell me that someone just prophesied over her that she was going to Russia.

Days later, I was sitting in my niece's back yard. We had just completed a memorial service for my brother-in-law Jim. My husband's cell phone rang, and it was Darlene. Pastor Alma, are you willing to go to Ukraine? I said yes. So, during the year of 2006, plans were being made for us to go minister in May of 2007, to women in Ukraine. I knew in my heart that one other person on our worship team was also to go. I asked her, and Cindy said, "Sister Bemis, call it done!" We began fund raisers to raise the necessary funds to take the trip. Gary e-mailed me to encourage us to take a male covering for every four women going. I asked my husband if he would be that covering.

Here it is January of 2007 and I am at McGee Hospital and doctors are telling me I may have fourth-stage cancer. I never lost the desire to minister to those women in Ukraine. I can't even imagine what some of them had gone through. When I would think about Chernobyl and the radiation that was released in the atmosphere over those people, I thought, just maybe, I will be an inspiration to someone. From the very beginning, I would ask the doctor's if I could go. At the start when they had set up the original plans of treatment, they were encouraging about the trip.

Now, I didn't know what to expect, I just had to take one day at a time. Yet, I remembered…"You are going to hear things you won't like, but trust me." My desire for Ukraine grew in my heart. I was determined to go.

They tried the needle biopsy, but were not able to get the tissue needed. They had to call in a surgeon to go in surgically to my lungs. When he came into the room, he explained that it looked like there where possible signs of cancer in the lymph nodes of my neck also. He said that he was going to go into the neck first. If there was cancer there, he would not have to go into my lungs. He said that they would keep me under anesthesia while they checked out the tissue, and only go in my lungs if that tissue proved negative. My husband was getting concerned because the surgery was taking longer than he expected, but then he remember, they will only go into the lungs if the lymph nodes were not cancerous.

The Calhouns, a couple from Pittsburgh, who often visit our church when they come to visit their daughter in Erie, were sitting in the waiting room with my husband. God has his family everywhere. They were such a blessing to my husband during this time of waiting. This is also the time the one nurse had come into pre-op, kissed me and told me she was praying for me.

The reports came back…no cancer in my lymph nodes and no cancer in my lungs. In both locations we were dealing with inflammation.

So now we are continuing with the first plan of treatment. I was going to return to Erie's Regional Cancer Center, and receive 25 radiation treatments, and five heavy doses of chemo-therapy. Then I would return to Pittsburgh for five internal radiation treatments. Before the treatments were completed two

Engraved

additional radiation treatments were added to deal with a lymph node in my groin area.

It was a Sunday morning, and often during the service my husband will feel lead to pray for people. This one particular service he called me forward to pray for me. He began to speak that the radiation and chemo would do the job they are assigned to do, and nothing more. I heard him, and couldn't believe he didn't pray for my healing. I didn't want radiation! I didn't want chemo! I wanted a healing. The Lord spoke to my heart: "Alma, no one likes radiation or chemo..give them to me." I knew He was dealing with my pride. I was quiet going home, and then began to share with my husband what I was going through. He began to apologize, and I told him that it wasn't necessary. I knew the words that he spoke were from the Holy Spirit, and I knew that God would walk with me through the treatments. I would lie on the radiation table, about to receive laser beams to four different locations of my body, and I would say, "Thank you Father that you are my shield." I never forgot the words my husband spoke that day. I stand in agreement with him that the two types of treatments would not destroy anything in my body that they were not designed to destroy.

The chemo specialist went over all the possibilities of what could happen. (You don't want to know!) He was then going to double check back with me about the dosage the doctors in Pittsburgh prescribed. He called me at my home and told me, 'You will definitely lose your hair." There were times when I was washing my hair that I would see more hair than normal on the shower floor, but I would begin to thank God that He had ever hair on my head numbered. Then I would remind the enemy that he would have to return anything that he had stolen from me. I never lost my head of hair.

The people at the Regional Cancer Center were incredible. The thing that broke my heart was the number of people having to deal with cancer every day. I was blessed because they have discovered anti-nausea medicine to take during and two days following chemo treatments. Those pills cost $100 each…but everyone going through the treatments are grateful for them. Though I had lost some of my appetite during the treatments, the main struggle was often dealing with either constipation or diarrhea. With God's grace, I made it through.

My brother-in-law Don died just before Easter from cancer. He was having trouble with reactions to his treatment. I would talk to him on a regular basis, and he would express his peace with God, and his love for me. I was so grateful that I got to Florida to spend time with him during the Thanksgiving holiday. I knew many people, with our being in ministry, whom had gone home to be with the Lord, while dealing with cancer. One of the greatest gifts that many of them have passed unto me is peace. I think of Irene Krantz, David Battistella, Judy Emser, Connie Verel, Tim Kuntz, Tracy Ross, Donald Covert, Mrs. Shea, Debbie Pernice and others who have gone on before me, but with faith and assurance that to be absent from the body is to be present with the Lord. I have known others that have had complete healings like

Mrs. Rozell, Marian Nellis, Marianne DiChristopher. Why one person lives and another dies, I don't have the answer to. Only God knows the answer to each and every person's destiny.

The whole process of my treatments was taking longer than I first expected, and I was to get on an airplane for Ukraine on April 29th. When plans were being made for the internal treatments, I asked the doctors again about my trip. They must have thought I was crazy! The first reaction was, 'No way!" The second thought was, we don't know how you are going to react to the treatment…let's wait to see how you do. The funds were non-refundable at this point, so that was not the issue.

I was scheduled to go for internal radiation treatments on April 16th. On Easter Sunday I got really sick. We were invited to my husband's sister's home for dinner. I told my family to go without me. I also told them I would contact them if it got worse. I was in so much pain; I had to be taken to the emergency room. Was I ever grateful for drugs at that moment, because at home I couldn't take even a sip of water without vomiting. I had done so well. I couldn't figure out what in the world was going on.

I told John and Cindy Morrison, a couple from our church, who were with me and my husband in the emergency room that God, had a reason for me being here. After many tests, one of the things that was determined was my white blood cells were extremely low. They would not have been able to do the internal treatments without them going up. I told the chemo specialist at the cancer center, and he gave me a shot to build the white cells up. I had the shot on Friday, and started internal radiation on Tuesday. God knew what I needed to go forward. Tuesday morning would have been too late to discover the problem. I would have never gone for help, if I could have taken a pain pill at home. God still works all things together for good to them that love Him, and are called according His purposes.

Now I'm in Pittsburgh, laying flat on my back for three days while 19 needles are inserted into the tumor. It is an incredible procedure. Every needle has a number, and is connected to a corresponding cable when you go for a treatment. They are able to control the amount of radiation going into each needle from the control room. Of course I am numb from my waist down during the entire time. On April 19th., they took the needles out, and I asked, "What about my trip to Ukraine?" The doctor said, while throwing his hands up in the air, "With your spirit, GO!" Ten days away, and we would be on our way.

When I had thought about what I was going to share at first, I thought it was important to discuss the first piece of armor that you must put on according to Ephesians 6. It is the belt of truth. None of the rest is effective without it. Your breastplate of righteousness is easily compromised without truth. Your helmet of salvation is weakened without truth. There is no way under heaven you can have God's peace without truth. Your faith can be easily shaken if it is not grounded in truth. Your shield will be hard to hold up without truth, and your sword can not ward of the enemy without truth. I purchased a white belt to take with me, as an object lesson when I spoke about it.

While I was in Ukraine, I was able to speak about the Lord being MY Shepherd. Psalms 23 became alive to me during this time.

(Psalms 23:1 NIV) A psalm of David. The LORD is my shepherd; I shall not be in want.
   (God has never left me empty during one trail of my life.)

(Psalms 23:2 NIV) He makes me lie down in green pastures; he leads me beside quiet waters,
   (During this time, I have had to do a lot of reflection and mediation of the Word.)

(Psalms 23:3 NIV) he restores my soul. He guides me in paths of righteousness for his name's sake
   (I have been made rich in the knowledge of who I am in Christ. He has helped me let of go of more things that needed to go out of my life.)

(Psalms 23:4 NIV) Even though I walk through the valley of the shadow of death, I will fear no evil, for you are with me; your rod and your staff, they comfort me.
   (Jesus is not a hireling that disappears on you when the wolf comes. No, He is MY

Shepherd! He never leaves me or forsakes me, and corrects me out of His love.)

Psalms 23:5 NIV) You prepare a table before me in the presence of my enemies. You anoint my head with oil; my cup overflows.
    (I can't wait to share more about the table in the next chapter.)

(Psalms 23:6 NIV) Surely goodness and love will follow me all the days of my life, and I will dwell in the house of the LORD forever.
    (I can't even begin to express the goodness and mercy that I have experienced day by day. I know that whether I live or die…I am His and He is mine.)

Engraved

What did I gain from going to Ukraine?

First of all I found a people of passion towards God. They had been suppressed under Communism for 70 years. Now they were passionate about their love for God and their call to minister that love to others. In Slyvansk I was so ministered to by them, I just wanted to sit in the presence of God and soak. During their time of worship, even though I did not understand the words, I knew the theme. Several times I would turn to my interpreter and ask what they were singing, and he would tell me. When he did, it was exactly what I was sensing in my spirit.

Second of all there is the need for the church to rise up and minister to the orphans all over the world. I was so thrilled to see the churches taking responsibility for orphans. They were teaching their people to adopt children. They had orphanages, yet the need remains so great. My husband was adopted as an infant, and he was able to share during the afternoon sessions about the affects of adoption on his life. Darlene grew up in foster homes, and was able to share what it was like to be a foster child. She was also able to share the affect of what a Christian foster home did to influence her life.

I was given the assignment of sharing with Pastor's wives. The very last day that I was teaching, I felt lead to share with them about pride. I told them my story of my husband praying for me the way he did. In the room for the first time was a Pastor's wife who had seven children. She had adopted four of them. As I was sharing the tears were coming down

Engraved

her eyes. I did not know that she was fighting the battle of cancer. I could just imagine the questions she had in her mind.

Earlier in the day, the Lord spoke to me to have three Ukrainian women pray for me that night after I shared my message. One was the Bishop's wife, one was Eugenia who coordinated the conferences, and one was the worship leader. After meeting this Pastor's wife who had cancer, I knew that I was to include her in the time of prayer. After I spoke about "The Lord is My Shepherd", I asked these three women to come and pray for both of us. The place went into a roar of prayer. As I knelt before them, I begin to weep over the love being poured out to our lives. When I lifted up my head flags were flying over us. I stood there and held this dear woman in my arms, feeling just about every rib in her body. Yet I know what she felt was love and acceptance being poured into her life.

One of the women asked me why I would ever choose her to pray for me. She was not worthy for such an honor. I told her she was worthy, not only to pray for me, but for others that God would put in her path. I get mad when I hear how little people think of themselves. I know that they have been fed a lie. God is calling us to reach out to one another in faith and love. The enemy wants us to feel like Christ in us means nothing. One woman came to me that was on the team. She said that she grew up in the church all of her life, but had never seen a leader humble themself in such a manner. She told me it had changed her forever.

Engraved

Back in Kiev, I had the opportunity to tour another ministry. It had a women's rehab center, and orphanage, a medical center, a training center, and a hospice center. When I came out of the training center, I stood against the wall and just said WOW!!! It wasn't about buildings, because their building wasn't great. It was about people having the passion to reach out to others.

Was the trip easy? No...but I will be always grateful the doctor said yes, and Darlene challenged me to go. It was something inside of me that I kept looking forward to in the midst of my storm, because I knew there was someone out there which had a need bigger than mine.

Engraved

Father:

How can I begin to thank you for Jesus, Your Son, and The Shepherd of my life? Not only does He walk through the valley of the shadow of death with me, but He enables me to partake of the wonders of love even in the presence of my enemies. He never leaves me. He never forsakes me. He is the glory and lifter of my head.

The Banqueting Table

The second week that I was in Pittsburgh, going through the test for my lungs, alone in my room, I found myself sitting in the spirit, at a table. To the right of me was Father God. I grabbed hold of His hand, then He grabbed hold of the hand of Christ, and He grabbed hold of the hand of The Holy Spirit. The Holy Spirit grabbed hold of my left hand. As this happened, I realized the love of The Father, the Passion in the eyes of Jesus, and the comfort and power of The Holy Spirit.

As I looked at Jesus, I asked Him if I could hold His hand. He told me that "I died and rose again so you could grab hold of The Father and the Spirit." "Every time you do, you become one with us." At that point, I knew what He desired when he prayed in John 17.

(John 17:20-21 NIV) "My prayer is not for them alone. I pray also for those who will believe in me through their message, that all of them may be one, Father, just as you are in

me and I am in you. May they also be in us so that the world may believe that you have sent me.

People began to come to my room, but the Lord told me to return later, because He wanted to show me more after the people had left. I went back to the table and took hold of the hands again. He showed me that the problem with a lot of Christians is that they grab hold of God, but when they leave His presence; the enemy is waiting with his hands outstretched. What is he waiting with? He hands out fear, poverty, riches, anger, pride, prejudice, discord, worldly pleasures, greed, and so much more. When we grab hold of anyone of those things as he offers them, we are becoming one with him.

I don't know about you…but I certainly do not want to become one with the enemy. I want to shake off anything that is not like God. So what do you do when the enemy wants to stretch out his hand to you? When you receive an evil report and fear is an option? You have to go back to the banqueting table and grab hold of God. Let Him speak into your life, through the Word.

I had to return to Pittsburgh for check ups and biopsies to see how I was doing. The doctor called me at home and told me that he was encouraged because the biopsy taken in his office came back negative. They were also encouraged because the tumor had shrunk. I was to return Friday for additional biopsies under anesthesia. When I received the next report it was that all but one biopsy came back negative.

Engraved

That one positive report meant that I would probably have to have radical surgery. Boy, I tell you the battle to grab hold of the wrong hand was raging. Radical surgery meant that I would have to have my bladder, vagina, and rectum removed. I had a choice to grab hold of fear, or grab hold of God.

The next day, I was going to attend The Tabernacle, in Orchard Park NY. Benny Hinn was going to be there, and we were going to have a homecoming celebration with him. My husband had been on staff at The Tabernacle for 29 years. It was my home church for 35 years. Benny use to come to The Tabernacle at least once a month when his ministry was starting out. This was sort of a family time.

I have to be totally honest with you…I was numb. I was just told that surgery was probably my only option for a cure. The last thing in the world I wanted to do was go into that service without faith. I didn't want people not seeing a woman of faith. I wanted faith written all over my face. I just wanted a moment alone with Benny…to say Benny I have faith. Yet, Benny couldn't give me what I needed. The service was incredible. Benny was sharing about worship. He began to share about John 17. I saw my banqueting table, and I saw Jesus being lifted up. All I wanted to do was worship Him. The Lord spoke to my heart and told me it didn't matter if Benny knew if I had faith or not…God knows what's in my heart. I had to return to His table, eat from His Word, and stand in His promises. I highly respect Benny Hinn, and I also know enough about him that his desire is that I would be in the face of God every chance I got.

As I continued to do so, my faith became stronger. I had to return to Pittsburgh for additional biopsies, and Pet-Cat Scan. The exact same results occurred, but I returned to the table, the Word, and His promises. I knew I was now strong enough to say NO! The doctor urged me to come as quickly as possible to have the surgery. I told him there was a time a person had to stand on their faith. His response was something like this; Mrs. Bemis you have been standing on your faith since day number one. I have seen people with less severe cancer die, because they had no faith. You have come through all that you have gone through with flying colors because of your faith. I believe you will make it through the surgery. I would think to myself, it doesn't sound like a healing to me, and the Word of God says, that "by His stripes I am healed." I would now tell the enemy he wasn't going to get another part of me. The more I spoke it, the more I knew I was doing the right thing.

One of the hardest things I had to deal with is that I knew the doctor was doing the best he knew to do. I knew in human understanding he believed there was no other way. The Bible says in;

> *(Prov 3:5-6 NIV) Trust in the LORD with all your heart and lean not on your own understanding; in all your ways acknowledge him, and he will make your paths straight.*

He was, through his training, fighting for my life. He was kind, and at the same time trying to convince me of the urgency of the matter. We had two telephone conversations about it, and after each time, I had to sort through all that had been said; then I had to build myself back up in the Word of God.

(Mat 4:4 NIV) Jesus answered, "It is written: 'Man does not live on bread alone, but on every word that comes from the mouth of God.'"

(John 6:35 NIV) Then Jesus declared, "I am the bread of life. He who comes to me will never go hungry, and he who believes in me will never be thirsty.

That is what is so important about the banqueting table. When I go to the Bread of Life, I have the strength to walk in joy.

I think one of the roughest weeks I had was when I began to focus on the looks in peoples eyes, and listen to the words of their mouths. I had to hear from God if I was going to conquer what I was feeling. He had me read about Joshua and Caleb. They were two of the twelve spies that went into Canaan to check out the land of promise, after Israel came out of Egypt. Joshua and Caleb came back believing the promises of God. The other ten spies came back and spread fear and unbelief. Because of the fear and unbelief, the children of Israel had to spend another 40 years in the wilderness. The only two of the older generation that would go into Canaan was Joshua and Caleb. During those forty years can you imagine the looks and the words from their generation that was dying in the wilderness? These two men had to put their focus on preparing the next generation for victory. Reading the Scriptures, and allowing God to speak to my heart, set me free from the looks and words of men. Now when it happens, I just say to myself, "Get over it, it's not 40 years."

I know the banqueting table is a place where I can go at anytime. I know that the seat that I sit in is my seat. I know that I will be fed from the Word. I know that when I leave I will be filled, but I also must be mindful to guard my heart and mind, because the enemy will do anything he can to trip me up. When he got done tempting Christ in the wilderness the Bible says in

(Luke 4:13 NIV) When the devil had finished all this tempting, he left him until an opportune time.

Yes, he is waiting for an opportune time. A time when we think we stand, a time when we are exhausted, a time when we least expect it. He wants us to turn and worship him, instead of worshiping God. He wants us to become one with him. He wants us to mistrust God, to question His promises. But the Bible says.

(Isaiah 40:31 KJV) But they that wait upon the LORD shall renew their strength; they

shall mount up with wings as eagles; they shall run, and not be weary; and they shall walk, and not faint.

Father:

How can I possibly express my gratitude for every Word that proceeds out of your mouth? You tell us that they that hunger and thirst after righteousness shall be filled. I know that you led me to the doctors I have, but I also know that they are only a part of the answer…you are the Great Physician.

(Psalms 107:20 KJV) He sent his word, and healed them, and delivered them from their destructions.

Thank you for sending your Word into my life.

Today

—⟁—

Good morning Alma. <u>Today is a day of victory, wonder, and glory; victory because the enemy is defeated, wonder because of who you are in Me, and glory because I will be the glory and lifter of your head.</u>

One of the most important things that I read in Dodie Osteen's book, "Healed of Cancer", is how she and her family came into agreement that if she believed she was healed; she should walk in that healing every day. She would not be babied by herself or her family. Dodie was sent home with fourth stage cancer.

I have the above first paragraph on my refrigerator to remind me that each and every day is an opportunity for me to walk in victory, wonder, and glory. I know that today opportunities will come my way to declare what I believe through what I do, and say. I don't want my life to stop because of the valley. I want to be fruitful in the valley.

When I first found out about the cancer, I was concerned on how it would affect my son Todd's goals for the near future. About five months earlier he came to us and told us that the Lord had been speaking to him about his future. He knew his long range goal was to go to Asia as a missionary. In order to do so he asked if he could move in with us if he sold his home. The second part of his goal was to move to Florida, and focus on his debt and further schooling. I did not want the cancer to change his moving to Florida in June. (Part of me would keep him by me forever...but the other part wants him to become all he is designed to be.) One of my first prayers was that it would not hinder his choices to go forward.

I received a phone call from Pam Grove, who is a local Pastor's wife. I had not talked to her at all in over a year, other than to say," Hi!" at a Faster Pastor Race at the Erie Speed Way. She told me she had a dream about me, and wondered if I minded if she shared it with me. I told her to feel free to share it. She told me that in the dream she was driving to my home, and there was great darkness all around it. When she got to my door there was a huge guard at the door. He would not allow her to enter my house unless she identified who she was. When she came in, I was in my pajamas, and my house was filled with peace. She said the strangest thing about the dream was that the guard was like a sumo fighter. I chuckled and knew the sumo guard represented Asia. I shared the dream with Todd and Maria, and told them to continue to go forward with peace. God would take care of me. That is exactly what the enemy wants us to do. He wants us to be paralyzed rather than walking forward with the plans of God for our lives.

In May:
I went to The Ukraine.
Came home and rocked my new-born granddaughter in the night.
We took a young girl from India, to visit successful Christian from India, in the Cleveland Area.
Spoke with my husband in Baltimore at a Pilipino Church.

In June:
I helped move my son to Florida.
Helped my husband sand hardwood floors we found in two bedrooms.

In July:
I had a picnic at my home for the women from our church.
Helped our new children's Pastor with their move.

In August:
I went to Cleveland to visit Mike after having his heart transplant. Praise the Lord!

In September:
We celebrated Pastor Reid's birthday, by going to Canada with him and Wanda.
We also went to the Pocono's and hiked at Bushkill Falls with our cousins Ruth and Bill.

Went to Sight and Sound to see "Creation."

Attended a Women's Conference in Lancaster, PA area.

Had Pastor Kelly and Mark Miller for the weekend.

In October:

I hosted a men's breakfast at the church.

Entertained Eugenia from the Ukraine.

Shared with my husband at three services in Buffalo.

Spent the evening with my sister in the emergency room.

Spent time with Maria's family celebrating the baptism of their new granddaughter.

Had a baby shower at my home for a woman having her first baby at 42 years of age.

In November:

We had a wonderful Women's Night Out, celebrating the influence other women have had in our lives.

Had the wonderful opportunity of having our India family of five from New Jersey visit for a weekend.

I had my mother-in-law move in for the winter.

We flew to Florida to spend Thanksgiving with our children.

Went to the Holy Land Tour.

We spent two days at Disney with Heather, Mom, Todd, and Jacob.

In December:
Todd, Maria, Jacob and Hannah were home for part of the celebration of the birth of Christ.

Why in the world would I even consider doing some of the things I did? Because I'm living one day at a time in victory, wonder and glory. I am careful to take a nap when I need to. My life didn't stop the day I found out about the cancer. Instead I choose each day to look forward to life. My husband just spoke a message on being fruitful in season and out of season. How appropriate for both of our lives.

Did my life slow down?...You bet it did...But did it stop?...NO!
Do I have my disappointments?...You bet I do... But they don't rule my life.
Have I shed tears?...Yes...But the joy of the Lord is my strength.
Have I needed to be held?...Yep...And my husband has wonderful arms.
Does wonder woman live at my house?...No... But God lives in my heart and mind.

I returned to Pittsburgh in October. It is the first time I saw the doctors since July. I was a little concerned about how they would be toward me, because of the choice that I made. I want you to know that they treated me with respect. I could tell by the look on the one doctor's face that he didn't know what he was going to find when he examined me. He was probably wondering how he was going to tell me

Engraved

---

what he found. Anyway, after three doctors examined me, they went out of the room to talk. The doctor returned with a different look on his face. They were surprised because the situation with the tumor was better, not worse. I shared with him that every time I prayed about the tumor, I did not feel that having the surgery was the right thing to do. I was standing on the Word. He told me that some doctors would drop me, but he would not. Then he encouraged me to continue to do what I was doing. A thousand pounds lifted off my shoulders, because he was willing to see me through this whole valley.

The other day while I was journaling, the Lord told me He was celebrating me. I asked Him what he was celebrating. He told me it was the truth that had been engraved in my heart and mind. The truth wasn't just someone else's story…it was permanently mine.

My Heart is Full Because:

I have a Peace that Surpasses all Understanding.

I have Grace Multiplied to My Life.

The Lord is MY Shepherd.

I have a Banqueting Table.

And Because of it, I Can Live Today.

Father:

Thank You for being a wonderful Engraver. My hearts desire is to know Christ more and the power of the resurrection. Thank you for every person who wrote a note of encouragement, said a prayer, made a dish of food, and helped clean my house when it was necessary. Thanks for giving people dreams, or words of prophecy. Thanks for the gift of faith. Thanks for helping me through the difficult times. Thanks for giving me a life worth living. Today is a wonderful day to be alive…because you fill my life with joy.

Engraved

By the way….

God gave me a new word to meditate on for 2008. The Word is "Wholeheartedness." He is teaching me so much about caring for this temple.

He gave me a Word	=	Wholeharteness
He gave me Instruction	=	"Getting Started on Getting Well" by Dr. Lorraine Day "Seven Pillaras of Health" by Dr. Don Colbert " Acid is for Batteries" by Dr. Victor A. Marcial-Vega.

He gave our church a $4,000 grant to teach our people to eat more fruits and vegetables, through the Body and Soul Ministries.

I will know when it is time to share more about it all…just know He's a Great Shepherd!